How to Lose Weight (And Keep it Off) By Reprogramming the Subconscious Mind

Lose Weight and Keep It Off By Transforming the Mind & Behaviors Volume 2

I0436443

ROBERT DAVE JOHNSTON

Published by:

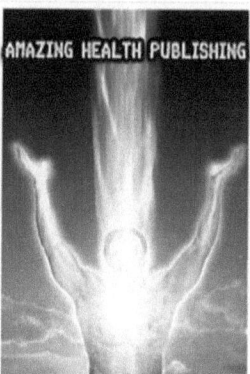

If you are interested in reading the next volume, follow Rob on Twitter @FitnessFasting

Copyright

Disclaimer & Legal Notices

The health-related information and suggestions contained in any of the books or written material mentioned above are based on the research, experience and opinions of the Author and other contributors. Nothing herein should be misinterpreted as actual medical advice, such as one would obtain from a Physician, or as advice for self-diagnosis or as any manner of prescription for self-treatment.

Neither is any information herein to be considered a particular or general cure for any ailment, disease or other health issue. The material contained within is offered strictly and solely for the purpose of providing Holistic health education to the general public. Persons with any health condition should consult a medical professional before entering this or any fasting, weight loss, detoxification or health related program.

Even if you suffer from no known illness, we recommend that you seek medical advice before starting any fasting, weight loss and/or detoxification program, and before choosing to follow any advice given this book. For any products or services mentioned or suggested in this book, you should read all packaging and instructions, as no substance, natural or drug, can be guaranteed to work in everyone. Information and statements regarding dietary supplements, products or services mentioned in this book many not have been evaluated by the Food and Drug Administration and are not intended to diagnose, treat, cure, or prevent any disease. Never disregard or delay in seeking professional medical advice because of something you have read in this book.

Nothing that you read in this book should be regarded as medical or health advice. If you do anything recommended in this book, without the supervision of a licensed medical doctor, you do so at your own risk. Not recommended for persons with any health related condition unless supervised by a qualified health practitioner.

Because there is always some risk involved in any health-related program, the Author, Publisher and contributors assume no responsibility for any adverse effects or consequences resulting from the use of any suggested preparations or procedures described in any of the books or other written materials associated with the website FitnessThroughFasting.com. The author reserves the right to alter and update his opinions based on new conditions at any time.

Dedication

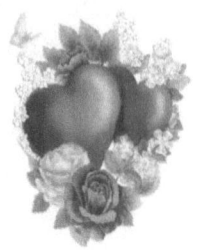

This series of books are dedicated to my mother Sonia Noemi, without whom I would not even be alive today. I love you mom. Thank you for never losing faith in me and supporting me, even when everything seemed hopeless and everyone else had given up on me. I owe you everything. I could collect all of the precious stones on this earth and lay them on your lap, and even still, I would not even come close to giving back to you all that you have given me.

Chapter 1: Unlocking the World Within

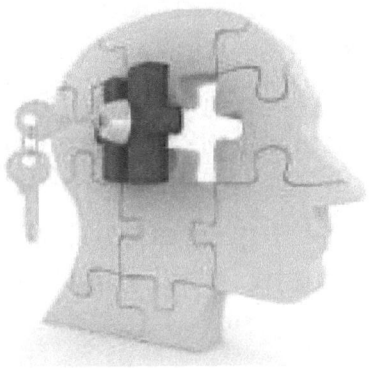

Many people fail at weight loss because they focus only on diet and exercise. Sure, these are important parts of the equation, but they aren't the most important. You can lose hundreds of pounds and look great. However, if you stop there and do nothing else, chances are that you will gain the weight back within a year's time *(or less)*.

Why? Because the inner world of thoughts and emotions was left unchecked. And if the old programming is not rewritten to support the new slimmer body, what do you think will happen? Yes, that's right... the mind will reshape the body in line with its existing unhealthy programming. How do I know this? I spent 20+ years trapped in obesity and binge-eating. Throughout the years, there were a few times when I managed to lose a considerable amount of weight. I dieted, worked out and was rewarded with results. But as the months went by, the weight always came back on. I was very frustrated by this see-saw of constant weight-loss/weight-gain. When I asked John, one of my mentors, what he thought the problem was, his response shocked me.

"Well," he said, *"you may have lost weight on the outside, but you probably still think and behave like an overweight person."*

John was once morbidly obese; he weighed nearly 500 pounds. He lost 345 pounds and had managed to keep it off for many years. So I was shocked by his response, but also quite curious. Over the following weeks, he helped me put together a personal inventory related to my thoughts, feelings and behaviors related to food. I was horrified by the results. Even when I lost weight, I still saw myself as a *'fat slob,'* which triggered anger and frustration which, in turn, led me to overeat and sabotage all of my efforts. It was as if my *'inner troll'* did not accept the thinner person in the mirror. That inner troll was fat, so it always rejected the slimmer man on the outside and used my thoughts, feelings and behaviors, to turn me back into its image. I realized that, if I wanted to lose weight and keep it off, I had to recreate the inner troll into one that supported the thinner, more active person that I wanted to be. That was a great "Ah-Ha!" moment for me. My personal inventory was full of statements like:

"You are fat and unattractive. You cannot control your appetite. You just can't help yourself. Nobody wants you anyways. Even if you lose weight, you're still ugly and undesirable. Food is the only thing that makes you feel good. You don't have what it takes to lose the weight and keep it off. You should just accept that you are obese and forget about weight loss. You're not strong enough to lose weight. You're weak... inadequate and pathetic. You're trapped. You'll always be fat. There is nothing you can do about it. Just eat and be merry. You're fat, but at least you're a nice person, so be happy with that."

And on and on and on. My goodness! How

on earth could I have possibly made permanent progress while being relentlessly bombarded with all of this garbage? It was a very painful but necessary realization. My initial discovery was this:

Long-term weight loss requires the development of a healthy belief system that supports it.

Otherwise, the weight loss-weight gain cycle continues, often for an entire lifetime. Until I 'reprogrammed' that inner fat guy, he would always sabotage my progress and revert my weight back to its distorted designs. Perhaps you already have proven this reality to yourself. If you have tried to lose weight in the past and have fallen short, then in this book I am going to give you some powerful tools that will **SOLVE THE PROBLEM**.

All I ask is that you keep an open mind and, more importantly, that you **roll up your sleeves and take action**. I don't write these books just to amass words on paper. I write them with the clear intention of **helping you to produce permanent results**.

And attaining permanent results will require some work. If you're willing to do the work to the best of your ability, then you can expect to see some very positive changes in the way that you think, feel and behave towards food and eating. What type of changes? Here are the benefits that you will gain if you give yourself wholeheartedly to this task:

- *It will become easier to resist temptation*
- *You will find yourself saying __NO__ to junk*
- *You will learn to manage and live with hunger*
- *It will be easier to make healthy food choices*
- *Exercising regularly will cease to be a struggle*
- *You will find yourself thinking and saying positive things about your body and appearance*
- *You will learn to the mind to 'Shut Up!" when the negative thoughts try to sneak in*

- *Your entire outlook on weight loss, fitness and health will be transformed - for the better*

I have experienced these benefits in my own life. And I have seen similar miracles come to pass in the lives of many others.
The bottom line is this:
  The only TRUE and LASTING change is the one that occurs from the inside out.

*Our external world is a mirror of our perception and belief systems. And, truth be told, **many people are viewing their lives through a very distorted and negative mirror**. This can be either conscious and/or unconscious.*

By identifying and correcting the lies and distortions, we begin to straighten out physically.

This is by no means an overnight process. It takes weeks and months of consistent work to start noticing the change in thoughts, emotions and, consequently, behaviors. But, if you are willing to be persistent, you will be amazed at the results. **Today can be the start of your own internal revolution.**

The time has arrived for you to overcome what has limited you; the time is **NOW** to lose the weight and <u>KEEP IT OFF</u>!

Chapter 2:
My Personal Hell

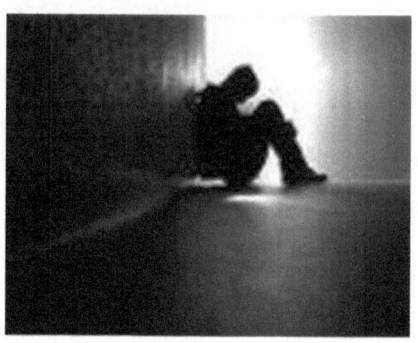

As I mentioned earlier, I spent nearly 25 years losing and gaining weight over and over... ad nauseam. The end result was always the same: obesity, binging, rage, frustration, self-pity, isolation and chronic depression. Being stuck in this vicious cycle - *as the years went by and by* - was one of the most painful and crushing experiences I've ever gone through. I felt like a bird trapped in a cage that was always covered, only darkness was my constant companion. It affected me physically, mentally and emotionally; everything seemed hopeless and, in various occasions, planned to take my own life. I recall feeling unworthy and inferior from the time I was a little boy. I was chubby and non-athletic. This made me easy prey for bullies; I was constantly pushed around and ridiculed because of my weight and lack of athletic ability. Most people that go through these types of situations outgrow them and become normal, responsible adults. I, however, found myself plagued by the same negative thoughts and emotions as an adult. These painful thoughts and emotions fueled my rampant binging, self-sabotage and destructive lifestyle. The *'inside troll'* was making sure that all of the negativity that I believed about myself became an **external reality**.

Sometimes these *(painful/negative)* thoughts, feelings and behaviors were conscious; I was aware of them, although I felt powerless to stop them. Example: *"I want to eat that pizza. I really shouldn't do it. It will undo all of the work you have done. What's the use? I'm only going to gain the weight back anyways! I might as well eat, be happy and accept my obesity. Yes, that's right."* And off I was to the pizza parlor to gorge and *'agree'* with the *'inner man's'* vision of who I was and what I should look like (fat). Other times, the wave of negativity was triggered subconsciously by external stimuli *(people, places, things)*.

Example: I would see a pretty girl and want to talk to her, but the *'inner troll'* would shout:

"She'll never talk to you! You're fat, ugly and nobody wants you! She's going to laugh at you and tell all of her friends. You're a born loser! She's way out of your league, forget about it! Now go eat a dozen donuts and that'll make everything alright!"

Whether the negativity was conscious or triggered by something external, I'd always end up binging to *'medicate'* the pain. Then the guilt, shame and remorse would strike without mercy.

I felt trapped and cursed to a life of obesity, isolation, depression and broken dreams.

Sure, I could lose weight; I lost dozens of pounds over the years. But my inner world remained tainted by pain, failure and misery (*nonstop negativity*). Inevitably, I would relapse into overeating and gain the weight back. After all, my mind told me that I was weak, fat, ugly, undesirable and unworthy of happiness. I learned to agree with the negativity and eat to feel better (*at least temporarily*). The destructive cycle solidified itself in my mind. No diet or fitness program (*alone*) could keep me thin because my thoughts, feelings and behaviors all supported the image of a fat, weak, '*loser*', that was ugly and undesirable. A mental trap of this sort is cunning and merciless; some people live their whole lives trapped in this juggernaut. It takes courage, commitment and patience to overcome it. And that's the good news: It **<u>CAN</u>** be overcome. I found a way out. And it consists of a **LOT** more than just dieting and exercising.

The first step was realizing that I had to "reprogram" my mind so that it would empower me rather than attack me.

Here the bottom line: The tools we're going to study helped me lose 90+pounds. Today, 11 years later, I have not gained it back. Sure, life is not Nirvana, and there are always challenges and struggles that we go through as human beings. But the chronic obesity, binging, depression and unhealthy lifestyle that kept me prisoner for all of those years have all but disappeared. And now it's **YOUR** turn.

Chapter 3:
Creators of Reality

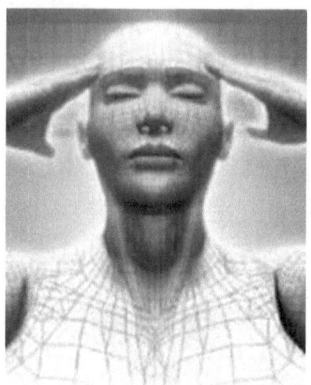

The foundation of the work we're going to do is based on <u>the power of positive thinking</u>. But let's define what I mean by *'positive thinking,'* because it is important for you to understand exactly where I'm coming from. Thinking positive is certainly nothing new.

In fact, the subject has been flogged to death in countless books, particularly in the past 30-40 years with the *'new age, new thought'* movements gaining popularity. The basic metaphysical concept is that <u>*'we are creators of our own reality.*</u>' That negative external **outcomes (including excess weight and poor health)** can - *in* *most cases* - be traced to negative belief systems and a distorted perception of reality. Let me illustrate what I mean when I say *'distorted perception.'*

The Mental Lens

You ever been to a circus or carnival and seen one of those funhouse mirrors that make you look really thin, and then really wide? Or, if you wear glasses that are dirty and smudged, how clearly are you able to see? If your camera had a dirty lens, how clear would the photographs be? That is what our *'mental lens'* is like.

The mental lens is basically the series of thoughts, belief systems and corresponding feelings through which we interpret reality and base our (positive or negative) life-philosophy and conduct.

I mean, if you read that last sentence several times, can you understand why this is so important? We're talking about your entire outlook on life! And, trust me, our relationship with food is a **HUGE** part of that general life stance. But, if the mental lens isn't clear, we will not see our life, future and possibilities in a positive fashion. This is the most insidious kind of self-deception that there is. We can be totally convinced that we are looking at *'reality,'* *(who I am, what I can or cannot do, my self-worth, my abilities)* when in truth, we're beholding a totally false and distorted perception of what is **REALLY** true.

What is the truth?

The *'truth'* is that **you are a worthwhile, unique and amazing human-being worthy of achieving all of your goals and leading a happy life. ANY** *(and I mean ANY)* thought, feeling and/or behavior that contradicts this truth is <u>false and distorted</u>. These must be identified, isolated and then *'reprogrammed '* through *'proper'* positive thinking.

Garbage In, Garbage Out

The basic premise of positive thinking is quite simple. To be sure, it is not hard to grasp the fact that *'what we put in is what we get out.'* Perhaps you have heard the expression **GIGO: Garbage In, Garbage Out.** So, by all means, I am a believer in positive thinking. The problem is that, over the years, the term *'think positive'* has, in many ways, become a joke. If all I had to do was *'think positive,'* then surely I would not have spent 25 years binging, obese and suicidal. When I hear someone tell a person who is depressed to just *'think positive,'* I cringe. Such a remark seems to suggest that, if only the person exercised more mental control, all of his or her problems would dissipate. No. That is **NOT** the type of positive thinking that I believe in. Such frothy emotional appeal is totally useless, insensitive and - in my opinion- insulting.

True positive thinking, in my opinion, must have a plan and strategy.

It must have a structured method that can be followed long-term. Just *'thinking positive'* sporadically *(without plan or structure)* does not work. So I want to make it very clear to you that, if you truly wish to attain results, you will need to commit yourself to a structure and follow it long-term. This is not about *'pop psychology'* or giving you a *'nice'* pat in the back. My aim here is nothing more and nothing less than **TRUE** transformation and **PERMANENT** change. If you can understand this distinction and are willing to do the work, then we are ready to move forward.

Chapter 4:
Self-Talk

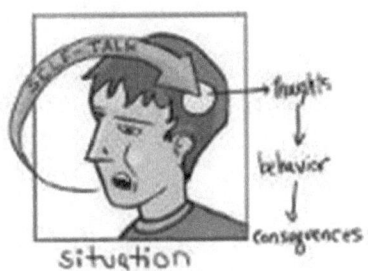

The best method I've found to implement *'true positive thinking'* is what is known as *'self-talk.'* Self-talk is exactly that: **the ongoing conversation that we have with ourselves, sometimes audibly but mostly silently in our own minds**.

We are constantly talking to ourselves and reacting *(emotions, conduct)* to this internal conversation.

Learning to control self-talk through a structured program of positive thinking *(as we are studying here)* **is one of the best tools available to make drastic (*and fairly quick*) changes in our belief system and behaviors.**

The problem is that most people live their lives without paying much attention to what they are telling themselves. As it relates to food and eating, it is no different. I have discovered that most people who struggle with their weight are plagued by negative self-talk; *"you're fat and ugly, you're no good, nobody wants you etc."*

So, in essence, self-talk constantly directs the course of our lives - good or bad. You may have *'caught'* yourself talking to yourself at certain times; at home alone, in the shower, while driving, standing in line etc. You may, in fact, be very much aware of your self-talk. You may freely admit that you are prone to negative thinking and that you often speak harshly to yourself. Those precisely are the patterns that I want to help you overcome as they have a direct (*and detrimental*) impact on our relationship with food and eating Even if the self-talk is only *'slightly negative,'* it still can interfere with the quality of your life and keep you from living to your fullest potential. And this ongoing self-talk, to a great extent, is fed by the volumes of information stored in the subconscious mind.

Chapter 5:
The Subconscious Mind

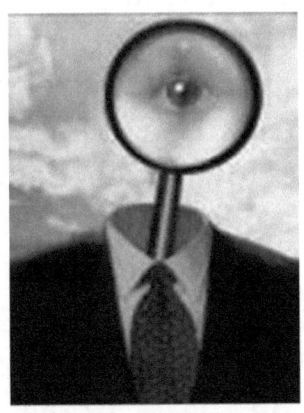

The subconscious mind is the part of the brain where all of your life experiences are stored. This includes memories, life-experiences, what you believe, what you like and not like, your outlook on life, skills you have learned, and pretty much everything you have heard and seen since you were born.

That's a **LOT** of information but, believe me, the human brain can more than handle it. **Our amazing brain has an estimated one billion neurons**, each of which connects to more than 1,000 other neurons - totaling connections in excess of one trillion.

To illustrate: if every neuron could only hold one single memory, then brain capacity would not suffice for a full lifespan. However, since the neurons in our brain work in unison with one another, they can *(collectively)* store around 2.5 petabytes of data. What the heck is a petabyte? One million gigabytes! How much data is this exactly? If we had a personal computer with this type of capacity, we could easily store in it <u>three-to-four million hours of movies</u>. If you wanted to watch all of the movies back-to-back, you would have to sit around watching TV for around 300 years! I hope that gives you an idea of the immensity of what we're dealing with here.

And the subconscious mind runs on 'auto-pilot,' meaning that a lot of this information is constantly being processed without any conscious thought whatsoever.

Automatic Subconscious Triggers

When a person is new with computers *(or any other task not done before)*, the learning process may appear daunting and insurmountable. Sometime later, however, the skill is mastered and the person can use a computer without much thought involved.

The person, in fact, can be using a computer and having a side conversation at the same time. The conversation is happening at the conscious level, while the computer-related functions are carried out by the subconscious, stored as a skill. The subconscious mind *'frees'* the conscious mind so that the latter can focus on other tasks and functions, usually of immediate relevance like chatting, cooking, reading a book etc. Can you imagine if every time you got in your car you had to think about how to drive it? If you've driven for some time, then you likely get in the car and drive away, right? The driving skill is *'stored'* in the subconscious and the information is used automatically and without effort. Another good example is that of breathing. When do we ever have to think about how or when to breathe? The subconscious mind runs that function as well.

Ego Defense Mechanisms

In addition to tasks like, walking, driving and using a computer *(among many others)*, the subconscious mind is responsible for automatic emotional surges that crop up when we're faced with challenges and uncertainty. A good illustration of this kind of subconscious emotional trigger are the jitters that most of us feel right before speaking in public or having to perform at any capacity. It is normal to suddenly feel anxious, nervous, fearful etc. After the activity begins, however, the conscious mind takes over *(giving the speech or performing the given task)* and the emotional trigger subsides.

Therefore, **just like the physical body has its own defenses against injury, so does the subconscious mind have protections from emotional wounds.**

These are known as *'ego or unconscious defense mechanisms.'* This <u>egoic</u> mechanism is there to guard you from emotional injury and to help you overcome them. The problem is that, in many cases, these so-called *'defenses'* end up hurting more than helping by *triggering all types of negativity that can keep you repeating unproductive behavioral patterns.* Furthermore, the subconscious mind also controls the logic center of the brain which solves problems, evaluates options, assesses outcomes and any other logical function that takes place while we're awake. This is the *'sixth sense'* or *'intuition'* which gives us a deeper evaluation of what we're dealing with at the time, and it also suggests options.

The Collective of Life Experiences

While emotional and logical triggers have distinct functions, they have one key element in common: **They are very much based on collective life experiences and personal belief systems stored in the subconscious mind**.

That means that, if the information stored is painful, negative, self-defeating, then the automatic responses triggered by the subconscious will end up creating more pain, misery and confusion. These are the automatic triggers that result in much of the negative self-talk that we discussed earlier.

Everything that we say to ourselves is influenced by the subconscious mind to a certain degree.

The mind cannot contradict itself. If the subconscious mind has stored the belief that "*I am a failure*," then it will be hard to live from a position of winning and being successful - **UNLESS** that rotten seed is identified, isolated and overwritten.

Chapter 6: Reprogramming the Subconscious

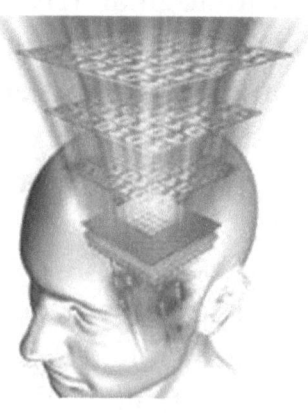

When information is absorbed and written into the subconscious mind, it becomes a basic program - very much like the software that you may run in your computer. As mentioned earlier, the information stored consists of everything you have seen and heard in your lifetime.

And since these programs are triggered automatically, then **the quality of the program being run becomes gravely important.** You wouldn't want to run a program on your computer that contained a virus, would you? Of course not.

However, most *people never take time to identify and heal the negative patterns in their subconscious minds*. That means that the negative, counterproductive programs 'installed' in the subconscious get to run around unbridled like a wild mustang, causing great havoc in people's lives. Then they ask themselves:

"Why can't I reach my goals? Why doesn't my life work? Why am I always so angry, unhappy, and sad? Why do I have to be overweight? Why do I eat so much when I know I'm not hungry? Why do I lose weight and gain it back?" And on and on and on.

But **THERE IS A SOLUTION**. And that solution is:

Reprogramming the Subconscious Mind - wiping out the virus and replacing it with a new (positive) program that supports rather than sabotages your life and goals.

This kind of reprogramming is absolutely imperative to repair the personality problems that keep you from losing weight and keeping it off. So was the case with me and many others. And so it shall be with

31

you, **IF** you are willing to do the work. Here's my point: *We need to have minds that help us reach our life goals, not make our lives miserable with automatically-triggered trash.*

Repetition, Not Logic

One of the most important points I have learned over the years is this: **The subconscious mind cannot be 'reasoned' with.** It will not respond to logical arguments as, for example, a persuasive conversation. To reprogram these subconscious patterns, we need **repetition**.

Studies in the science of persuasion indicate that **a logical argument won't always work, but you can usually change a person's mind if you repeat the message over and over.** That is a huge clue for us who want to overcome negative subconscious patterns. It tells us that giving the mind reasons why it should think this or do that won't work.

However, giving it a *mantra (repetitive message)* over a period of time **WILL** work and cause the new message to be absorbed. The conscious and subconscious minds can work together and do amazing things if all of the negative garbage is taken out. Working to create this balance is one of the most important things you could ever do for yourself.

Creating positive, useful cooperation between the conscious and subconscious minds will sharpen your learning capacity and give you the ability to master your emotions. And, as we know, emotions are one of the key triggers for binging, nibbling, overeating, eating between meals and so on. So, as you can see, there is a direct correlation between reprogramming the subconscious mind and losing weight and improving eating habits.

We have the ability to reprogram our mind and give it direct and to-the-point directives that support the goals and lifestyle that we want for ourselves.

I must admit that at first I thought all of this mind programming stuff was hogwash, silly and totally a scam. John would present the program to me and I would scoff. "*I hate that new age crap,*" I'd say. He would simply smile and say, "*That's alright. You'll hit a bottom.*" Then he'd walk away.

And he was right; the ongoing emotional pain, coupled with more demoralizing binging and weight gain, softened my resistance. I became willing to try it with an open mind. The results have been life-changing and led me to write this book you are now reading. Now I am passing it over to you! Let's get started.

Chapter 7:
Affirmations

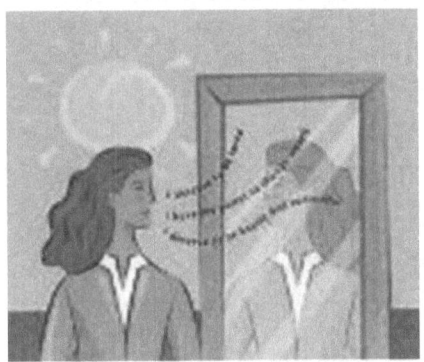

The most powerful way to use positive thinking to reprogram the subconscious is through affirmations. You probably have heard a lot about affirmations - positive **statements about something you desire to become and/or accomplish.**

Affirmations can be done by writing them down *(around 50 times each day)*, writing them once and then reading them aloud to yourself *(at least three times daily)* or recording the affirmations and then listening to them daily. Or a combination of the three. Our work together will focus on the latter two. Overall, the goal of affirmations is to **give the subconscious mind direct and positive commands,**

repeated with conviction and strength. Affirmations are a way for us to 'coach' or own minds. Imagine that you have a good friend who wants to accomplish a goal that he or she thinks is beyond reach, like, for example, running a marathon.

Since you care about this person, what would you do? Would you tell him or her to forget about it, that they'll never win... to give up, go home and hide under a blanket? Or would you motivate them, tell them to keep trying, to not give up? I am certain that you would do the latter. You'd want to fill the person with positive words and encouragement, right? Well, that is exactly what affirmations do. The difference is that, with affirmations, we are giving that same support to ourselves.

How often do we treat ourselves in ways in which we would <u>NEVER</u> treat another person? I know that I can be very harsh with myself. Perhaps you can relate.

Affirmations help to program the subconscious just like code is used to program a computer. We repeat the words and focus on the goals we want to reach, forming mental images of us accomplishing the objective. Affirmations, in essence, open the door to **creative and positive visualization**.

How Long Will It Take To See Results?

As I have explained, this entire *'reprogramming'* process must have a structure. The reason why most people fail when trying to reprogram their minds is because they do it *'whenever and however'* and **do not have a firm plan of action that they commit to long-term**.

We are very impatient beings. We want instant results! And if the results do not materialize overnight, then we become frustrated and convince ourselves that *'this doesn't work.'* I know because I did that myself for a lot of years. The key is commitment and persistence.

Ok, Robert... but how long will it take to see results? For many, the changes are quick and drastic... in a few days they start to notice that their attitude is changing.

For others, these results could take weeks or months. For me, to be honest, it took close to 3 months to **REALLY** notice marked changes in my personality. It all depends on how committed you are to seeing the process through and how thorough you are in following my instructions. I am going to serve it all to you in a gourmet plate. But you still have to dig in and do it.

What are the changes that you can expect to notice?

- You will notice that you are much calmer; things will not get to you as much as they used to.
- If something made you really emotional before *(in a negative way)*, you will find yourself <u>not</u> reacting as much.
- You will find it easier to <u>not eat</u> in between meals. You may feel hunger or cravings, but **you will find the inner strength to say no and wait until it is time to eat**.
- You will find yourself willing to go to the gym more often.
- The amounts of food that you eat will decrease.
- You will want to be more active than before... and so on.

The changes will be quite noticeable. I want you to understand, however, that **you must**

have a deep desire to change the way that you think... period. In this book, we are focusing on weight loss. However, the changes you make <u>here</u> will impact <u>every other area of your life</u>. It will be important for you to become the *'watchman of your mind.'*

No longer can you allow the mind to run to-and-fro like a wild horse. If you allow that, then the results will take much longer to materialize.

Commitment and persistence are an absolute must.

Chapter 8:
Into Action

STARTING TODAY, DO THIS:

1. Go to your local pharmacy and purchase a package of flashcards.

2. Fill at least 20 of them with positive affirmations about your weight, health and self-image.

3. Write in the present tense so that your subconscious mind absorbs the statement as a *"done deal"* and not a *"pie-in-the-sky"* far- flung wish distant in the future.

Here are some examples from my personal collection:

- It is <u>now always</u> easy for me to control my appetite <u>at all times</u>.

- It is <u>now always</u> easy for me to say no to *(list your specific trigger foods)*. Mine was pizza and donuts.
- I <u>now</u> lose weight easily and effortlessly <u>at all times</u>.
- I <u>now always</u> have supernatural will power to achieve <u>all</u> of my goals <u>all of the time</u>.
- It is <u>now always</u> easy for me to keep the weight off and I <u>always and easily</u> resist <u>all</u> temptation.

Evaluate the different areas of your life that you wish to change and form statements directly related to them. These can include self-esteem, spirituality, lifestyle etc...
For Example:

- I <u>now and always</u> feel great about who I am and am <u>constantly</u> filled with intoxicating passion for life <u>at all times</u>. **(Self-Esteem)**
- I <u>always</u> receive powerful spiritual guidance and discernment to overcome <u>all</u> problems <u>at all times</u>. **(Spiritual)**

- I <u>always</u> am filled with energy and motivation to live and love to be outdoors and active <u>at all times</u>. (**Lifestyle**)
- It is <u>now easy</u> for me to talk to others and I <u>always</u> feel great about myself <u>in every situation</u>. (**Social**)

You can, of course, add your own. Once you have them ready, pull them out in the morning <u>in a quiet place</u> and read them to yourself out loud. Allow each word to enter into your mind. **Imagine the message penetrating into the center of your soul**.

If you receive negative inner feedback like: *"Yeah, right! Poppycock! These are lies; you're weak and you'll never make it! This is stupid. This doesn't work, you're wasting your time!"*

Just let the thoughts pass and continue. That *'inner troll'* that we talked about at the beginning will fight for his life. He will see that the new statements will eliminate his dominion over your mind, so it will resist in many ways, particularly by invalidating your efforts and telling you that everything you are doing is worthless. Being aware of this subterfuge will help to keep you going. No matter how loud and aggressive the inner voice gets, continue to read the cards. Over time, you will notice that the resistance will diminish. Eventually, it either disappears altogether or becomes but a minor irritation.

<u>The bottom line is this</u>:

The mind <u>MUST</u> eventually adhere to the directions you give it!

If you follow a specific religion, end the session with the prayer of your choice and whatever other inspirational material you are accustomed to reading. Repeat the process during the day when the mind starts to fill you with negativity, fear, worry, doubt or unbelief. Anytime you are tempted to nibble, binge or eat between meals, take out the cards and read through them, aloud if possible. I carried my pack of flashcards in my pocket for months and months. It was my most precious lifeline.

I never left home without them. **I knew that if I went back to where I came from I was dead**. So I clung to the flashcards as a child would his favorite safety blanket. It was very hard to drive by donut and pizza shops because normally I would pull right in and eat compulsively. It was very hard. But when the moment of temptation came I would promptly pull out the cards and read them. **This interrupted my negative impulses and centered me with positive reasons for <u>NOT</u> giving in**. So do it. Do it, do it, do it! Culminate the day by doing a final reading immediately before going to bed. Make sure that the very last message your subconscious receives is a positive one.

Now, Always & All the Time

Take notice of each of the words I underlined in the above affirmations: **always, now, at all times** etc... Why did I highlight them? Those questions are giving the subconscious mind <u>clear instructions of what we wish to happen</u> <u>NOW</u>, <u>ALWAYS</u> and <u>ALL OF THE TIME</u>.

I want your subconscious to receive a new program that automatically triggers positivity for you now, always and all of the time.

Remember, the subconscious cannot be reasoned with. It will simply go on the information that you give it. If you say <u>NOW</u>, it will say, *"Ok, great... let's do it now then*." If you tell it <u>IN EVERY SITUATION</u>, then it will take it literally and produce the results as commanded. So, yes... it is <u>VERY</u> important that each of the statements you write have those key words in them. Use them in whichever way you want, but make sure to use them.

Do this detailed exercise consistently for two weeks. Work the flashcards until they wear out in the corners from your thumbs. Make sure to do the readings three times daily without fail - rain, shine or sleet. This will serve as the '*appetizer*' for the main course, which is moving on to **Recording the Affirmations In your Own Voice**.

That may initially sound corny and silly. It certainly did to me. In fact, John had his hands full with me because I refused to do it. I thought it was the stupidest thing ever. But, let me tell you, I eventually came around.

Chapter 9:
Are You Ready For the Transformation?

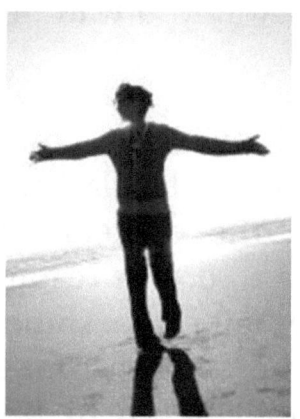

Getting Started

Once you have laid the foundation with two solid weeks of reading the flashcards (*at least*) three times daily, you are ready to move on to Phase II.

DO THIS:

If you have a cassette recorder, purchase new batteries and buy a pack of 90- minute cassettes. You can buy them cheap at any pharmacy. Or, if you have the hardware on your computer to record audio and own a CD player, then purchase some **blank**

rewritable CD's with at least <u>700</u> <u>megabytes</u> of storage space. These, too, can be purchased at any pharmacy for about $10.

->

Select a time in which you can be on your own, undisturbed.

Turn off your cell phone and television. If you do not live alone, **let others know that you do not wish to be interrupted for at least one hour**.

By the way, you **DO NOT** have to explain in detail to <u>anybody</u> what you are doing. In fact, I would recommend that, *apart from a very select few,* you do not trumpet to everyone what you intend to do. Many persons simply will not understand and are likely to criticize or even ridicule your efforts. This can even happen with members of your own family. **So be careful**. You do not need any more negativity. Lord knows, we sure have enough in our own minds, right?

Now, find some type of soothing music that you can integrate to the background. I would recommend instrumental music. You don't want your mind distracted by lyrics. Mellow, **instrumental meditation music**

is best, but make sure to use music that really inspires you.

Inspirational music can open your subconscious mind to receive the message, and also produce positive emotional reactions that can be <u>attached</u> or associated with the new messages.

Sit down and get ready to start recording. Make sure you find a comfortable chair.

Chapter 10:
Making the Recording

You are now ready to start recording. If you are using a cassette player, do some test recordings to see which distance from the microphone produces the best sound. Do the same if you are recording on the computer.

Make sure there is no echo or static that affects the clarity of the recording.

<u>You want each command to be heard clearly and up front</u>. The music should be in the background, also, so make sure that it is not too loud.

When all looks good and you are ready, press record and begin. Each affirmation you use will be recorded in both the "**I**" **and** "**You**" tenses.

I'll explain why in a minute. To make it easier for you, below is the list of affirmations that I recorded for myself. Pay attention to the words that I underline and remember what I explained earlier about why it is important to emphasize them.

1. It is <u>now</u> <u>always</u> easy for **ME** to control MY appetite <u>at all times</u>.

   (Say your first name) It is now always easy for **YOU** to control your appetite at all times.

2. It is <u>now</u> <u>always</u> easy for **ME** to say no to **(fill it in with your specific trigger foods)**.

   *(Say your first name)*It is <u>now</u> <u>always</u> easy for YOU to say no to **(indicate types of foods that you want to avoid)**.

3. I <u>now</u> lose weight <u>easily</u> and effortlessly <u>at all times</u>.

   (Say your first name), **YOU** now lose weight easily and effortlessly <u>at all times</u>.

4. I <u>now and always</u> have supernatural will power to achieve <u>all</u> of **MY** goals <u>at all times</u>.

   (Say your first name), **YOU** now<u> and always</u> have supernatural will power to achieve <u>all</u> of **YOUR** goals <u>at all times</u>.

   Think about the different areas of your life that you wish to improve, and record affirmations directly

related to them. These can include self-esteem, spiritual, lifestyle...etc.

5. I <u>now and always</u> feel great about who I am and am <u>always</u> filled with intoxicating passion for life <u>at all times</u>.

   (Say your first name), **YOU** <u>now and always</u> feel great about who you are and are <u>always</u> filled with intoxicating passion for life <u>at all times</u>.

6. I <u>always</u> receive powerful spiritual guidance and discernment to overcome <u>all</u> problems <u>at all times</u>.

   (Say your first name), **YOU** <u>always</u> receive powerful spiritual guidance and discernment to overcome <u>all</u> problems <u>at all times</u>. **(Spiritual)**

7. I <u>always</u> am filled with energy and motivation to live, and I <u>always</u> love to be outdoors and active at <u>all times</u>.

   (Say your first name), **YOU** <u>always</u> are filled with energy and motivation to live and **YOU** <u>always</u> love to be outdoors and active <u>at all times</u>.

8. It is <u>now</u> <u>easy</u> for **ME** to talk to others and I <u>always</u> feel great about **MYSELF** in **every** situation <u>at all times</u>.

   (Say your first name), It is <u>now</u> easy for **YOU** to talk to others and **YOU** <u>always</u> feel great about **YOURSELF** in every situation <u>at all times</u>.

<u>Note</u>: I <u>strongly</u> recommend you **take your time and draft your own**. If you did the previous *"flashcard"* exercise, then you can simply transfer those to the audio tape. But, believe me, the more you do it, the more affirmations you will suddenly come up with to address other thinking patterns you want to change. I initially came up with ten basic statements.

However, each day I would think of a new one and, eventually, I made a recording with around 40 statements like the ones above. So please don't rush through this or take shortcuts writing the statements. Add to them regularly and dig deep into the mind to find more and more directives. Once you have finished recording, stop and review what you have done. Great job ... but there is more.

Chapter 11:
The Power of Your Voice

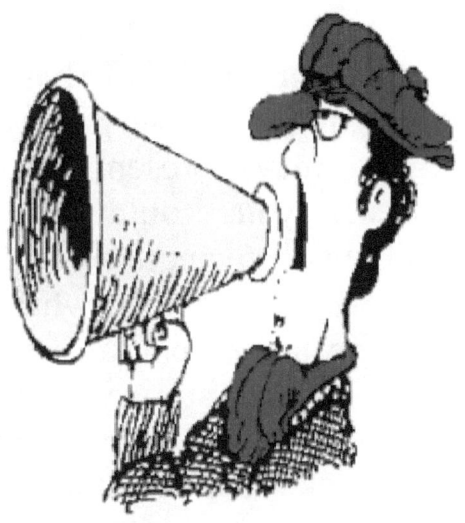

Why this insistence on making the recording with "**I**" and then "**YOU**"? Well, when we talk to ourselves, most of us use both of these tenses. Spend a day listening to and taking notes on your "*inner talk*" and you'll see what I mean.

For that reason, doing affirmations in both **I and You** hit both sides of the equation *(conscious and subconscious mind)* and maximize the impact of these powerful statements. When you first start to hear your own voice on the recording *(talking to* *yourself)*, you may feel silly, stupid or even spooked. All of this is perfectly normal and will pass after a while. **Do not let that stop you!**

You may even get angry and feel that you are wasting your time. It is very possible that your mind may present strong arguments as to why you should **NOT** do this, and why all this *"affirmation"* stuff is garbage and useless. Remember what we said earlier about the *'inner troll's'* resistance and how it will try to stop you from overwriting its presence in your mind. I went through a heck of a mental battle when I first began.

The negative programs in the subconscious mind will *'fight'* to survive. If you've never done something like this, you are giving the subconscious a **HUGE** shock. So initially it may resist via strong emotions <u>AGAINST</u> this work.

At one point I destroyed the audio recordings and threw my journal and flashcards in the trash. However, I was so fed up with the that way I was living, I was so thirsty for something better, that I reconsidered and re-recorded the statements. I am very glad I did.

Don't let any resistance you feel at first keep you from taking action.

Little by little, you will become more and more receptive to the messages and start to welcome them. New visions of yourself will start to open up and, over a period of weeks, you will notice subtle changes in your mood and attitude.

Specifically as it relates to binging and overeating, the biggest impact comes when the "*voracity*" to eat (*the wrong foods*) starts to diminish. Suddenly it isn't such a horrible battle to eat clean and not nibble.

<u>The bottom line is this</u>: *your mind knows who you are. It recognizes your own voice and sees it as the ultimate authority. Sort of like the child who immediately reacts when he or she hears the voice of a parent.*

So begin to <u>parent</u> your own mind. **Give it specific directions of what you want it to do and how you want it to function**. The mind can be like a wild horse that, if left unchecked, will buck violently and throw you to the ground. But, once you assume the authority that is rightfully yours, you will notice that **it will obey and actually be glad that some "adult" with sense has finally shown up! One more thing**: When you record, use an <u>assertive</u>, <u>forceful</u> voice. Not violent, but rather **firm and to-the-point**. This is no time to whisper or speak meekly. **Let your mind know that you mean business. Do not be afraid to use strong voice tones**.

Put all of your passion and emotion into each statement. I got into it so passionately that, when I finished, I was drenched in sweat and actually felt a little hoarse. I felt angry at all of the limiting thoughts and belief systems.

I was fed up of wasting so many years of my life in anger, sadness and disappointment. When you are finished, you should have a minimum of 30 minutes worth of "**I and You**" statements directly linked to the changes you wish to make in your life.

Chapter 12:
How to Use the Recording

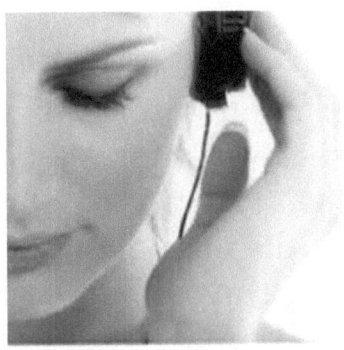

My suggestion is that, if possible, you take the CD or cassette with you and listen to it while you are out.

When you have a break - *like when having lunch* - put on some headphones and listen to the recording. Observe your reactions and journal them. **What answer does the mind give you**? For me, the reaction was usually something like:

"Baloney! You're a loser; you'll never make it, you might as well give up!" Also, gauge your emotions.

One technique that worked really well for me was to wear the headphones at night while sleeping. Let the recording pound the subconscious all night long. That is a very good time since, while we sleep, the subconscious is much more active - hence dreaming.

The subconscious mind absorbs everything that it hears even as we sleep. When I first started doing this, I recall having some amazingly- vivid dreams about success, traveling and being surrounded by light. I am pretty sure that listening to the powerful statements while sleeping had a lot to do with that.

Chapter 13:
Breaking the Chains

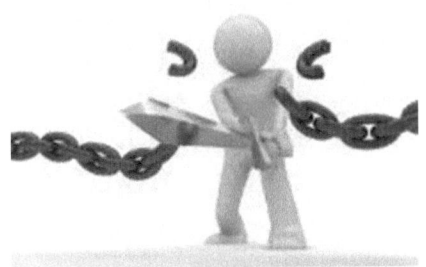

Everything we have been discussing comes down to one thing: **Personal Responsibility**. Life waits for nobody, and time continues to pass for us all.

You can either let your mind and circumstances victimize you and lead you further and further away from your dreams and goals, or you can take action and do whatever is at your disposal to improve the quality of your life.

Indeed, it is never easy to get started. Especially when one is overweight and has been that way for a long time. So, while at first it may seem like an uphill battle, I tell you that **you are worth it**. It <u>WILL</u> get easier. Considering the option of doing nothing and getting worse, **whatever price of discomfort and frustration you pay now is little in comparison to the ultimate price of sickness and unfulfillment.** Pay the price **NOW**. Take action. Be persistent. Do not **EVER** give up! So, as I always like to say: **Easy Does it - But Do It!** Seize the challenge, walk through it, and allow it to transform you into a stronger and healthier person. You can do it!

If Nothing Changes, Nothing Changes

My primary message to you is this: **DO NOT** start fasting, dieting, and/or exercising while allowing the mind to just sit idly. Make sure that, while you are working hard to improve your physical body, you also are cleansing the mental garbage. Give your mind a constant feeding of powerful, direct and to-the-point thoughts that push you forward.

The mind WILL respond and you will notice amazing changes in your behavior and the way you think.

I'm sure you have heard the expression: "**If Nothing Changes, Nothing Changes.**" You can lose all of the weight that you want and become ultra-thin and sexy. But if there were no *"inner"* changes in the way you think, then it is very likely that the mind will sabotage your progress. Please, please... I beg you. Do **NOT** let this happen to you. Don't take this message lightly.

I learned many years ago that "**Freedom Carries Sacrifice**." Losing weight and having optimum health are both very important goals.

But to maintain it long-term, it **is imperative to directly and forcefully address those internal voices that attempt to destroy our dreams.**

Chapter 14: Assignments

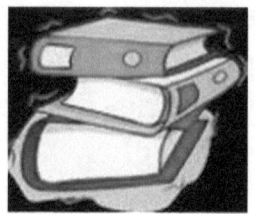

1. **Read This Material Several Times Until You Fully Internalize the Material**: At first glance the mind may tell you that what we are discussing here is petty and silly - and that it will not work.

   If you *"react"* to this, then you will have closed the mental door and the principle will not work. So be persistent. **Be open minded**. Read this book slowly and thoroughly. Give your mind and heart <u>time to absorb and internalize what is being said</u>.

2. **Take Immediate Action and Carry Out <u>ALL</u> Of The Directions Outlined**: Make a commitment with yourself to follow through on what we have discussed here <u>**IN SPITE**</u> of any negativity or protestations your mind may give you. If you *"don't feel like it"*... <u>do it anyways</u>. **Get up! Now!** Get the flashcards and sit down

to put together your list of positive statements. Do not procrastinate... don't leave it for tomorrow. *THERE IS NO TOMORROW!*

Remember, by doing this you are standing up to negative belief systems at both the conscious and subconscious levels. So **be prepared for resistance**. In fact, **look at resistance as a clear-cut sign that you are moving in the right direction**.

A salmon does not become discouraged and turn around when it swims against heavy current. It keeps going <u>undaunted</u> until it reaches its destination. Do the same! Do the *"flashcard phase"* of the assignment at least three times a day for two weeks. The best times are upon rising and before retiring... once in the middle of the day is also recommended to keep negativity in check.

3. **Move On To The Audio Recording Phase**. Take the statements that you wrote on the flashcards and put them on audio with some soothing instrumental background music. You do not have to turn this into an elaborate recording either. A cassette deck works just fine. Make it easy on yourself.

This is your private self-improvement project. Nobody else needs to be listening to the recording. Just do it. If you prefer to do an mp3 and download it to your portable player, I recommend the **Audacity audio recording software**. It's free and very simple to use. All you need is a microphone and you're ready to go. If you have a webcam, then chances are that it has a built-in microphone. If not, you can go to a discount store and buy a web microphone for around $20.

4. **Switch to Reading the Flashcards at Least <u>ONCE</u> Per Day (rather than two or three), and - instead - Listen to The Audio Recording <u>AS OFTEN AS YOU CAN</u>.** Keep reading the flashcards when you wake up in the morning, and take the audio with you and listen to constantly through the day. Listen to it in the car, listen to it while in line at the bank, listen to it in the toilet, listen to it while eating lunch *(given that you're alone!)*, and - last but not least - **LISTEN TO IT WHILE YOU SLEEP!**

5. I usually put on the recording while I'm falling asleep. I usually wake up at around 3 or 4am to drink water. At that point I

remove the earphones and go back to bed. So I'm not saying that you HAVE **TO** keep the audio going **ALL** night. You can, by all means, but if you do it for several hours each night that would work great.

6. **Start A "LIFE JOURNAL" and Write About Your Goals Related to Weight Loss, Health, Food and Eating.** Make it a point to write on your new journal **DAILY**. Whenever the urge to eat the wrong foods comes, spend some time writing about what you are thinking and feeling. Nine times out of ten there will be fear, anxiety or boredom. Feel the feelings without having to always *"medicate"* with food.

You will be amazed when the urge to eat goes away and you see that you **CAN** do this. I want nothing more than for you to experience this freedom for yourself. There is nothing like it!

Write about any mood swings and make sure to jot down the reasons why you want to lose weight and get healthy. The whole point is for you to constantly *"remind"* yourself just how important it is for you to see this process through ALL **THE WAY!**

7. **Communicate with A Person or Persons Close To You Who Know That You Want To Lose Weight and Improve Your Diet and Health.** While you do not want to trumpet it from the rooftops, it IS a good idea to have some type of personal accountability. Find somebody that you trust who will support and not judge.

Talk to that person frequently, especially when you find yourself struggling. Moreover, I strongly encourage you to form an online support group of people to share your health, weight loss-related goals.

Please do not isolate or try to do this alone. Go to FitnessThroughFasting.com and enter Fasting Forum #1 or Forum #2, and post messages. Ask for support. Read other people's posts and reach out! You will find many people on the same path. You may even make life-long friends!

8. **No Matter What Happens In Your Life, Stick To Your Flashcards and Audio Assignment For One Year.** Make it a priority to assault your mind with these statements **FOR A FULL YEAR** and do not let anything or anyone detour you

from this path. Do it daily. Do it constantly. You will be in for some very profound changes in your outlook and behavior. As I said, there really is no excuse for **NOT** doing this. You have nothing to lose and EVERYTHING to gain! So let's go... get started today!

Until next time...
God bless and Godspeed,

ROBERT DAVE JOHNSTON

Dear reader: Thank you so much for reading this book. If I can be of further service to you in any way, you can write me at: webmaster@fitnessthroughfasting.com
Hang in there and never give up! May rich and wonderful blessings overflow in every area of your life, and in the lives of your loved ones!

Grab The Entire Collection:

Volume 1: The 'Permanent Weight Loss' Diet

Volume 2: The Intermittent Fasting Weight Loss Formula

Volume 3: How to Lose 30 Pounds (Or More) In 30 Days with Juice Fasting

Volume 4: Lose The Belly Fat Fast, And For Good!

Volume 5: Lose the Emotional Baggage: Transform Your Mind & Spirit with Fasting

Volume 6: How to Break a Fast (or Diet) and Keep the Weight Off

Volume 7: Compilation Volumes 1-6 -> Get All 5 For The Price Of 3!

Also by Robert Dave Johnston:

How to Lose Weight & Keep it Off by Transforming the Mind & Behaviors

Volume 1: How to Build a Rock-Solid Foundation That Supports Long-Term Weight Loss

Volume 2: How to Lose Weight & Keep it Off By Reprogramming the Subconscious Mind

Volume 3: How to Beat Diet Hunger and Junk Food Cravings

Volume 4: How to Escape the Diet "Time Trap" and Succeed in Weight Loss

Volume 5: How to Cheat on Your Diet (And Get Away With It)

Volume 6, Compilation: All 5 for the Price Of 3

Also By Robert Dave Johnston:

Detoxify Your Body, Lose Weight, Get Healthy & Transform Your Life

Volume 1- The 10-Day 'At Home' Colon Cleansing Formula

Volume 2- The 30-Day Kidney, Parasite & Liver Detox Weight Loss Method

Volume 3- Lose Weight Fast & Detoxify With Intermittent Fasting & At-Home Coffee Enemas

Volume 4 - Compilation: Get All 3 For The Price Of 2! Detoxify Your Body, Lose Weight, Get Healthy & Transform Your Life - Volumes 1-3

Don't forget to check the articles and growing health community at: FitnessThroughFasting.com